Intermittent Fasting

The Superior Lean Muscle Building and Fat Burning Secret for an Enjoyable Lifestyle

not allowed unless with written permission from the publisher. All rights reserved.

The information provided herein is stated to be truthful and consistent, in that any liability, in terms of inattention or otherwise, by any usage or abuse of any policies, processes, or directions contained within is the solitary and utter responsibility of the recipient reader. Under no circumstances will any legal responsibility or blame be held against the publisher for any reparation, damages, or monetary loss due to the information herein, either directly or indirectly.

Respective authors own all copyrights not held by the publisher.

The information herein is offered for informational purposes solely, and is universal as so. The presentation of the information is without contract or any type of guarantee assurance.

The trademarks that are used are without any consent, and the publication of the trademark is without permission or backing by the trademark owner. All trademarks and brands within this book are for clarifying purposes only and are the owned by the owners themselves, not affiliated with this document.

Introduction

Thank you and congratulations for buying this book, *"Intermittent Fasting: The Superior Lean Muscle Building and Fat Burning Secret for an Enjoyable Lifestyle"*. Here you'll read about the amazing benefits of this eating schedule and how to implement it to improve your health and lifestyle.

Fasting isn't a new concept. In fact, fasting has been a part of different cultures all over the world. People tend to fast for health, spiritual, or religious reasons. You must be wondering what intermittent fasting is all about. It is an elementary concept. Intermittent fasting is a particular pattern of eating that oscillates between periods of eating and fasting. This is quite different from other traditional diets. It helps in cutting down on the overall consumption of food without leading to a severe calorie deficit. Picture this, you skip your breakfast and then have two hearty and healthy meals within an eight-hour feeding window (let's say 12 pm to 8 pm). Does this sound awfully simple? Yes, it is as simple as that!

Do you feel full after eating or do you start craving for something else? Would you like to control your irregular hunger pangs? Do you want a diet that isn't restrictive like other diets? Do you want to lose weight or maintain your weight loss? Well, if your answer is yes to the above-mentioned questions, then intermittent fasting is the right diet for you. This is one of the most flexible eating protocols ever and doesn't take much extra effort to follow. Depending upon your lifestyle and daily routines, you can select a fasting method that fits the bill.

In this book, you will learn about the different variations of intermittent fasting, the various benefits offered by this eating schedule, how to get started with intermittent fasting, about exercising on this diet and will find certain tricks and strategies to make sure that your body adapts to it successfully.

This book contains a wealth of information about this practice, which has had so much publicity in recent times.

If you are interested in intermittent fasting, then this is the book for you! We can step into the world of intermittent fasting. Are you ready to shake things up in your life?

Table of Contents

Chapter 1: What Really is Intermittent Fasting and How to Boost Its Results

Our ancestors didn't have the opportunity to eat three, four or five times a week. They had to hunt to survive and barely eat a portion of raw meat once a day. Think about it for a moment.

They survived and I can bet they neither felt starving all the time nor were obese at all.

So, what is fasting? The definition by itself is simple, fasting is the voluntary abstention from food. Fasting is different to *famine*, which is forced deprivation of the population of food and the resulting starvation, through natural causes such as crop failure, (one such instance occurred in China in 1958 as a result of an initiative of the communists called *The Great Leap Forward*.) Fasting is usually done for positive reasons, sometimes religious or spiritual. It is different to the self-imposed starvation, for very damaging purposes, of *anorexia nervosa*, a disease, usually associated with teenaged girls.

Intermittent fasting defines itself. Is as simple as alternating between the periods of fasting and the so called "feeding windows" periods where you can eat. Intermittent dieting does not specify any particular diet, such as ketogenic or paleo. Rather it emphasizes a pattern of regular alternation between fasting and eating. Some intermittent fasting methods split a day or week into fasting and eating periods as we will discuss in later chapters.

Most people have a period of fasting each day, as they sleep. All intermittent fasting does is extend that fast longer in different ways. As an example, one of these involves not having breakfast and consuming the first meal at midday and the last meal in the evening, at say 8 pm. The practice of intermittent fasting is quite straightforward and not difficult. It is a strange fact that a lot of people say they feel better and have greater energy while fasting in this way.

Only in the beginning you may feel hunger pangs. That does not necessarily mean hunger. Your body will start to get used to abstaining from eating for longer periods of time. We'll address this issue later in this book in a progressively manner.

How to Maximize your Results and Become a Fat Burning Machine

Intermittent fasting is an effective way to shed all those extra kilos and maintain the weight loss on its own. However, if you want to speed up the process of weight loss you can combine this eating schedule with a powerful and proven diet.

Ketogenic and Paleo diet are the most common for accelerated weight loss. They are not subject of this book but let's give them a quick look.

A ketogenic diet (or "keto" for short) is a high fat and a low carb diet. In this diet, the body makes use of ketones to producing energy instead of glucose and hence the name of this diet.

When you combine these, you need to just make sure that during your feeding window, the food you are consuming is keto-friendly, meaning that it has a high fat and a low carb content. Have lots of meats and vegetables instead of having carbs. Stay away from all sugary products as well. Naturally fatty foods like full-fat dairy products, meats and fish will leave you feeling full while reducing your calorie consumption.

On the other hand, Paleo diet is all about going back to our roots and eating the way our Paleolithic ancestors did. If our cavemen ancestors couldn't eat something, then neither can you. This is a high fat and a low carb diet also. It is mainly based on the consumption of whole and unprocessed foods.

If the food you eat matches with the keto or paleo aspects, then it will highly increase the far burning process in your body. So, why don't you try mixing things up a little and see for yourself?

Still skeptical? I understand. Most people react the same way the first time the heard about it but let's dive into how it works from a biological and scientific point of view.

Chapter 2: Why is Intermittent Fasting So Effective and How It Can Work for You

This chapter is short, but vital. Many people employ intermittent fasting for weight-loss. Weight-loss is only one of the many reasons for using intermittent fasting. Fasting is a potent therapy and has many benefits. You might think that the enforced deprivation of the body of nutrients while in a fasting period could cause damage and, it is true, especially initially, when the body is put under stress.

However, it is the reaction of the body to that stress that is the reason for the health benefits. This stress encourages the body to activate functions that repair and protect it. The processes by which the cells of the body divide and die is tidied up in a much more organized way when intermittent fasting is occurring.

It is typical of people leading modern lives to put their bodies under pressures that are alien to the way in which humanity evolved. By incorporating intermittent fasting into our lives, we can reap these benefits and guard against many of the ill effects that modern life can cause.

In addition to the promotion of weight-loss, fasting rapidly removes from the body excess sodium and fluids, eliminates the problem of *edema*, which is swelling in the body caused by excess fluid, and hence reduces blood pressure.

It benefits the body's sensitivity to insulin. Insulin is an enzyme produced by the pancreas and as a result of insulin sensitivity; the body absorbs glucose from the bloodstream in a healthy way, as an energy source. Without insulin, sensitivity, glucose builds up in the blood leading to diabetes and other serious health problems.

Fasting benefits all negative aspects of what is called *metabolic syndrome*. Metabolic syndrome is an umbrella term to describe a group of conditions: elevated blood sugar levels, excessive blood pressure, too much body fat near the waist, and unusually high cholesterol or triglyceride levels that often occur together. When they do there is a great increase in the risk of stroke, heart disease and diabetes.

By removing stored toxins, fasting is very good for detoxification. It enables the gastrointestinal tract to fix itself, which often leads to huge improvements not only with digestive problems but also in most aspects of health.

Fasting activates SIRT1 genes. These genes cause reduction in inflammation and in stress caused by oxidation and increase the survival of cells and hence promote longevity. This gene causes a chemical reaction called *deacetylation* in proteins that regulate cells. It is this process that is so helpful to the survival of cells.

Before finishing this chapter, the reader is reminded to seek prior medical advice before performing any form of fasting. Although fasting, particularly intermittent fasting, is quite safe, do not fast if you are:

(i) Pregnant
(ii) Breastfeeding
(iii) Under unusual stress
(iv) A child or teenager
(v) Suffering from anemia (too few red blood cells)
(vi) Suffering from a liver or kidney complaint
(viii) Training hard in a demanding strength sport like weightlifting, rock climbing or gymnastics

Even if you are in one of these categories, you may find that intermittent fasting is right for you but should seek professional, medical advice before embarking on it.

In the next chapter, we'll look at a whole list of benefits that you can start to experience rapidly as a result of implementing Intermittent Fasting to your life.

Chapter 3: 15 Health Benefits You Can Start Experiencing by Implementing Intermittent Fasting

As we mentioned above, there are many benefits from intermittent fasting, and they are not only related to fat-burning or fitness purposes. Some of these include anti-aging, brain functioning and more.

Let's see.

#1 - Weight Loss

The main reason that many people will take up intermittent fasting is to help them lose weight. Intermittent fasting, particularly when combined with a sensible exercise and a solid diet, is a powerful tool in the fight against the obesity epidemic that is sweeping the world.

Now, just in case it's not clear, there's another basic principle that must be in place for you to lose weight: caloric deficit. Eating ten thousand calories on your feeding window will just make you a disservice.

There are endless examples of people who have successfully lost weight and retained the lower weight when on a program of intermittent fasting. Sometimes efforts to reduce weight, even if they use intermittent fasting, are unsuccessful. There are many reasons for this such as hormonal imbalance, stress, poor sleep, and even prescription drugs. Despite these problems, intermittent fasting is a beneficial strategy for losing weight but if you find that you are unsuccessful, when intermittent fasting or otherwise, in the loss of weight then you may be well advised to seek medical help.

#2 – Sleep

In the paragraph above, it was mentioned that sometimes efforts to lose weight are undermined by insufficient sleep. There has been at least one scientific study, which has shown that people who persist with intermittent fasting for a year or more have a better sleep. The reasons why this occurs are no doubt complicated, but there have been conclusive demonstrations that intermittent fasting over an extended period assists good sleep.

#3 - Mood and Motivation

The study of the effect of intermittent fasting on mood and motivation is in its infancy. There is a lack of research on large populations, using the statistical techniques of randomized controls. However, there have been some studies, though, which have demonstrated that intermittent fasting does improve both mood and motivation in a surprisingly short period. As there is profound controversy about the pharmacological treatments of people's mental state any treatment, which has no side effect and many potential benefits must be considered seriously.

#4 - Resistance to Illness

In the previous chapter, there was mention of the positive role of intermittent fasting in the life and death of cells. Generally speaking, for lots of reasons, intermittent fasting improves the health of individuals and hence makes them more resistant to illness.

#5 - Cardiovascular Health

Intermittent fasting leads to a reduction in weight. For this and other reasons, it leads to an improvement in cardiovascular health. The cause of such disease is usually atherosclerosis, the deposit of plaque in blood vessel walls. The dysfunction of the endothelium, which is a thin lining of the blood vessels, causes atherosclerosis. A healthy endothelium works to prevent this insidious deposit. The endothelium is not doing its job properly if plaque builds up. Obesity, especially where the fat deposits are in the abdominal area, leads in many cases to this buildup of plaque.

Other causes of this deposit are stress and inflammation. Intermittent fasting assists in the reduction of these as well as obesity. Some studies show improvements in all risk factors for cardiovascular health.

#6 - Gut Health

Increasingly scientists are becoming ever more aware that microorganisms living in the human gut or digestive system perform vital functions. These are known as the *microbiome*. There are trillions of them and they are in other parts of the body, apart from the gut. Much disease originates in the gut, not only in that part of the body, but also of the brain, the heart, and all other regions of the body.

There is research on mice that calorie restriction improves that part of the microbiome in the gut. The effect of this is to prolong the life of the mice. In humans, the effects of dietary changes are very swift, even as short as hours. Studies are currently being done to verify that the real effects of intermittent fasting observed in the gut health of mice are true for humans as well.

#7 – Brain

Research has shown that the reduction in calorie intake of intermittent fasting has beneficial effects on the brain. Intermittent fasting results in something called brain derived neurotrophic factor (BDNF) that improves the means by which the brain neurons resist degeneration and dysfunction.

A consequence of intermittent fasting on the brain is that it boosts its power. The fasting triggers a mild stress reaction in the brain, which makes it more active. Scientists explain this by the evolution of the brain in prehistoric times, which conditioned it to become more active when food was needed.

Studies with rats have shown that intermittent fasting can prevent the onset of memory problems for times equivalent to at least 20 years in human beings. Study throughout the world to confirm that these positive results for intermittent fasting by rats apply for people who practice intermittent fasting.

#8 - Neurodegenerative Diseases

This term may seem a bit strange to most people but what follows may help. Two well-known neurodegenerative diseases are Alzheimer's disease and Parkinson's disease. Alzheimer's is a grave condition in which a person's memory is progressively destroyed with the illness usually being fatal. Famous individuals who have had it include the great US President Ronald Reagan and the well-known singer Glenn Campbell.

Parkinson's disease is also severe; it is a disease of the nervous system, whose symptoms include tremors and slow movements. It affects older people with the evangelist Billy Graham and the famous singer Linda Ronstadt having had it. Unlike Alzheimer's, Parkinson's, although debilitating, is not always fatal.

There is research to show that lowering the intake of energy by fasting often, at least twice a week, regularly, may assist the brain to avoid neurodegenerative diseases, such as Alzheimer and Parkinson's. Some may ask, 'Why not just reduce the amount of food eaten?' A smaller food intake is of less or no benefit because the glycogen stored as a result of this eating may not be used for up to 12 hours.

Eating three meals a day with snacks in between does not give the body the chance to deplete the resulting glycogen. Fasting is a way in which the body must practice autophagy (self-eating of cells). It won't do this if there is glycogen present as an energy source.

#9 – Diabetes

Diabetes, by itself, is a severe condition and is often a precursor to serious cardiovascular diseases such as heart attack and stroke. The cause of diabetes is the buildup of glucose in the blood. Diabetes occurs when the body is resistant to insulin. Intermittent fasting reduces the buildup of glucose (blood sugar) and substantially lowers insulin resistance. Intermittent fasting is an excellent protection against the onset of diabetes. Research has shown intermittent fasting to be beneficial for men in particular.

#10 – Inflammation

We are all familiar with the inflammation that occurs in throat glands when you have influenza or the inflammation around a scab as a cut heals. These inflammations are part of the body's way of dealing with real damage.

Unfortunately, not all inflammation is good; inflammation is often the cause of many serious problems such as diabetes, atherosclerosis and neurodegenerative diseases. This sort of inflammation is called *chronic inflammation*. It occurs when the body is unable to remove the source of irritation. Research has shown that the modern lifestyle with its excess sugar, processed food, chronic stress and lack of exercise is often to blame for chronic inflammation.

Researchers at Yale University have discovered that a compound produced by the body during intermittent fasting wards off the inflammatory response in many situations where it is not needed and could cause damage.

#11 - Autoimmune Diseases

These are quite common even though they are not as well known, as they should be. They affect about 50 million people in the USA alone and many hundreds of millions of others in the rest of the world. The cause is the body's immune system, which works to protect it against foreign intruders, turning on healthy cells in different ways. There are more than 80 autoimmune diseases; some of the most common are rheumatoid arthritis, celiac disease (gluten intolerance) and psoriasis, a skin condition, which affects many. Intermittent fasting has been shown to be beneficial to the sufferers of many autoimmune diseases.

#12 – Pain

As mentioned above intermittent fasting has proved to assist in reducing inflammation significantly. One of the benefits of this reduction in inflammation is a decrease in pain. There have been many reports of different sorts of pain reduction as a consequence of intermittent fasting.

#13 – Skin

One of the benefits of intermittent fasting is usually an improvement in the quality of the skin. The reason for this is that when fasting the body's cells has a reduction in the aging process. We shall have more to say about the effect of intermittent fasting on aging near the end of this chapter.

What about diseases of the skin? Research has shown that intermittent fasting had a very positive effect on 80% of the sufferers of psoriasis. Other dangerous conditions of the skin, which benefited from intermittent fasting, were contact dermatitis, acne and eczema.

#14 – Cancer

The very word cancer terrifies most people. There are many sorts of this disease, some far more virulent than others, and it is unlikely that there will ever be one single cure for all cancers. Although it is not a cure, intermittent fasting helps to prevent cancer. It contributes to reducing the very adverse effects of modern treatments such as chemotherapy.

#15 - Longevity: Does the idea of living to the age of 100, with a crisp brain, in real health appeal to you? Of course, it does; life is precious and is worth savoring. It has been conclusively shown, both with experiments on animals and observations on human populations that a reduced intake of food using intermittent fasting promotes a longer life. Why is this so?

Recall from the last chapter: *The processes by which the cells of the body divide and die is tidied up in a much more organized way when intermittent fasting is occurring.* Although no one knows exactly why intermittent fasting promotes longevity the effect of intermittent fasting on the cells will almost certainly have much to do with this.

Enjoying this book so far? I hope you have received some valuable information and I would LOVE to hear your honest feedback. Leave us a review on Amazon.com.

In summary, we can say that intermittent fasting, when combined with a sensible diet and exercise regime, will greatly assist in the quest for a longer, healthier and happier life. The benefits of intermittent fasting are the substance of the previous chapters; it is now <u>time to act</u> describe how to practice intermittent fasting.

Chapter 4: Five Different Methods of Intermittent Fasting for You To Choose From

As mentioned at the end of the last chapter, we now turn to the actual methods of intermittent fasting. As with many human activities, there are many ways of doing this and it is best if you find one that works for you. Here are some methods.

16/8 Protocol (a.k.a LeanGains): In this method, you fast for 16 hours then eat regularly during the next 8 hours. Since few of us get any nutrients while asleep, it is sensible to include the time spent sleeping as a part of the 16 hours.

Within this eating window, you can squeeze in two or three meals. This method is popularly known as the LeanGains method, and Martin Berkhan, a fitness expert, popularized it. This is one of the simplest forms of intermittent fasting. It can be something as simple as skipping breakfast and having your first meal at noon and the last one before 9 pm.

The fasting window in this method is restricted to about 16 hours daily. It is advisable that all the women who are interested in taking up this approach shouldn't let their fasting period go over 14 to 15 hours. If you are used to skipping your breakfast, then this method will be quite easy for you to follow. During the fasting period, you can have plenty of fluids, along with calorie-free beverages. So, you can have herbal tea, green or black tea, and black coffee! If you are keen on losing weight, then make sure that you steer clear of all junk and processed food. This diet will not work if you binge on calorie rich foods during your feeding window.

If you want to follow the LeanGains method of intermittent fasting, you will have to get used to fasting on a daily basis. The plan for this method is quite simple. Make sure that most of your fasting time falls within your sleeping period. You will have to fast from midnight until noon. Your sleeping and fasting periods will be between midnight and 8 in the morning.

Suppose you start your fast at 8 pm then you would not eat anything until 16 hours after that time which is 12 pm on the next day. Lunch on that day would be your first meal. You would be allowed to eat until 8 pm when the cycle would start again.

The same schedule will be repeated daily. The only time available for you to eat will be the eight hours where you are allowed to eat. You will be fasting for an average of 14 to 16 hours every day.

16:8 DAILY INTERMITTENT FASTING

Source: Dean Yeong of DeanYeong.com

You could tweak this same protocol to different timespans holding the same basic principle. Some practitioners use a 14/8 protocol, 18/6 protocol, a 19/5 protocol (The Fast-5 Diet) and even a 20/4 protocol which we'll discuss underneath.

The Warrior Diet: This is similar to the 12/8 and 18/6 methods. You could call it a 20/4 protocol. If you started fasting at 8 pm, then you could eat from 4 pm until 8 pm on the next day. The only refinement in this method is that you are supposed to have only one large meal in that 4-hour period. You may well wonder why you would do this. The answer given by the proponents of this method is that, by doing this, hormone production in the body is optimized and excess fat burnt, particularly if you reduce your intake of carbohydrates.

Ori Hofmekler popularized this diet, and he is a well-renowned fitness expert. This form of fasting involves the consumption of small quantities of raw fruit and veggies during the day and then consuming a single hearty meal at night. Essentially, you will need to fast throughout the day, and then you get to feast at night. The feeding window extends to only 4 hours. This variation of the intermittent fasting diet was one of the first ones to be popular. While following this method of fasting, the food choices that you make should be quite similar to what you would have made had you been following the Paleo diet. You will need to consume foods that are unprocessed. You can eat anything that our cavemen ancestors would have consumed.

1 Day Feast/1 Day Fast (a.k.a Alternate Day Fasting): As the name suggests, this diet is all about fasting on every alternate day. There are different variations of this diet. Some variations allow you to eat about 500 calories on every alternate day, and the others require you to observe a strict fast on every alternate day. Most of the lab studies that have been conducted to find the benefits of intermittent fasting have made use of some variation of this diet. A strict fast might sound rather severe and extreme. Depending upon your comfort level, you can adapt this diet to suit your needs. It is advisable that beginners don't immediately jump into this method. With this method of fasting, be prepared to go to bed hungry a few times every week. This diet doesn't show any form of sustainability in the long run.

This form of intermittent fasting requires the individual to fast for 24 hours, once or twice every week. Brad Pilon, a fitness expert, popularized this diet a few years ago. You will need to fast for 24 hours in this diet. From dinner on one day until dinner the consecutive day, that will constitute 24 hours. For instance, you had your dinner at 7 pm on Monday, and you don't get to eat until 7 pm on Tuesday. This would be the 24 hours fasting window. You can also do this from breakfast on a given day until breakfast on the following day. You will just need to fast for 24 hours; you can select the timings according to your convenience. You cannot consume any solid food during this fast. However, water, coffee and other beverages that don't have any calories in them can be safely consumed. If you are following this method because you want to lose weight, then in such a case you will need to eat regularly during your feeding window. You should eat the sort of food you are used to eating, had you not been fasting. The only problem with this method is that there happens to be a 24-hour fasting window and it might be difficult for a few people to follow. You don't necessarily have to start out with this. You can gradually progress from the 16-hour fasting model. The first stretch of the diet wouldn't be hard. It is only towards the end that this diet gets a little complicated to follow. This is where discipline and motivation will come in handy.

ALTERNATE DAY INTERMITTENT FASTING

Source: Dean Yeong of DeanYeong.com

5/2 Diet: This is a method of intermittent fasting, which has received a lot of publicity throughout the world. This promotion is due to Dr. Michael Mosley, a British researcher, who has led an extensive and public investigation of intermittent fasting, written up in the book he co-authored with Mimi Spencer called *The Fast Diet*. In this method of intermittent fasting, you eat, as usual, for three days then have a fasting day followed by two days of feasting followed by another fasting day after which the cycle repeats. On fasting days, you are allowed to eat food with a caloric content of about 500-600 calories.

The most liberal of all regimes is called the **Anything Goes Method** and says that you eat when your body tells you that you are in need of food. This method is not a sound idea for overweight people who are accustomed to massive intakes of food. The body will have hunger pangs, when in fact feeding as they normally do is not sensible, and those pangs ignored. This method is excellent for people with good self-discipline who have a healthy body weight and are only fasting for health reasons.

There is no structured plan for this form of intermittent fasting. You can reap all the benefits offered by an intermittent fast without having to plan any elaborate meals. This is quiet an easy variation to follow. You will simply have to skip meals spontaneously from time to time. Skip meals whenever you aren't hungry, or you are preoccupied with some work. It is a myth that people will need to eat every couple of hours. Your body won't start losing muscle or even shift into starvation mode if you go without food for a couple of hours. Our bodies have been designed in such a manner that we can go without food for prolonged periods of time. Missing one or two meals from time to time will not do your body any harm. In fact, it will give your body a break and provide you with an opportunity to cleanse it. So, if you aren't hungry, you can skip one meal. Then depending on your hunger quotient, you can have a hearty lunch or dinner accordingly. However, you will need to make sure that the other meals that you are consuming are healthy.

No matter which way you pick:

 (i) You should start slowly and not be in too much of a rush. On fasting days you should eat less than normal but don't starve yourself to the extent that you give up too soon.

(ii) On fasting days, particularly, if all you need is good health maintenance, you can have about 20% of your regular caloric intake on fasting days.

(iii) Drink plenty of water and other fluids such as soft drink (few calories), coffee, and tea, a small amount of milk in these drinks, if preferred, is harmless.

(iv) Avoid processed food as much as possible, particularly if the food has sugar in it. Most processed foods do in fact have a lot of sugar in them.

(v) No matter what method you choose, it will be much easier for most if their spouse or partner is supportive or even joins them in intermittent fasting.

(vi) Special occasions such as the visits of friends and relatives, Christmas, Thanksgiving, etc. may need you to sacrifice a few days of your regime. If you find that you have to do this, then don't worry about it. If you resume your intermittent fasting when the occasions are over then, there is no permanent harm.

In the next chapter will discuss other facets of your life that you need to apply or avoid to successfully accelerate the positive outcomes you so strongly desire.

Chapter 5: Other Facets of Health

This chapter looks at some other aspects of life, which are vital for overall health.

Do you need more than Intermittent Fasting for good health? The answer to this is an unequivocal YES. The list below is probably not exhaustive but includes many things you need to consider.

Exercise: Exercise is as vital to good health as is diet. You have probably heard this time and time again, to the point of being bored, however, it is true. There is an abundance of research proving the benefits of exercise. Like intermittent fasting, the only choice is which type of exercise you will do rather than whether you will do it.

Most experts recommend some aerobic exercise, such as running, cycling or walking for the lungs and blood circulation and some anaerobic exercise, such as weights or machines, for the muscles and bones. You may object to such a regime, citing such things as time and other commitments. Even if you do, you should always do some exercise and there are even exercise routines of only a few minutes, such as the Tabata method, devised for those who want their exercise finished as soon as possible.

Sleep: Good sleep is an essential component of a healthy life. Some people find it hard to sleep well. You don't have to sleep for a very long time every night. However, there should be at least two nights every week when you get a good 6-8 hours sleep. Although intermittent fasting can help you sleep better, there are occasions when sleep is hard to get. Things that you can do to improve your sleep include:
(i) Be sure to refrain from alcohol of any sort for at least two hours before you go to bed.

(ii) Try and get some aerobic exercise, preferably outside, such as walking or jogging earlier in the day.

(iii) Avoid the use of mobile phones, tablets such as iPads, and computers in the evening. The use of flickering screens is not conducive to a good night's sleep.

(iv) Avoid worry as worry causes stress.

Stress: Stress is the reaction of the body to challenges. Stress is beneficial if a crisis arises. Such stress is called *acute stress*. Stress, which causes massive problems is a different form of stress and is called *chronic stress*. Chronic stress results when the stress system of the body is continually stimulated and never has a chance to stop. It is important to learn to relax and to avoid taking problems to bed, doing so causes worry, which prevents sleep.

Sun: The skin weighs twice as much as the brain and is the barrier that protects our vital organs against the elements. For a long time, there was a widely held belief that a heavy suntan was healthy when in fact this was simply not true. The sun's ultraviolet rays, although important to our wellbeing in moderation as a source of vitamin D, among other things, can be very harmful. Nothing can cause damage quicker to the skin than over exposure to the sun. Protecting yourself against its ravages is imperative.

Smoking: Smoking is the number one preventable cause of adverse health in society. No industry has contributed more to human misery than the tobacco industry. The attitude of the entertainment industry in portraying smoking as a regular and glamorous activity is nothing short of a disgrace. You will undermine many of the benefits of intermittent fasting if you smoke!

Chapter 6: Intermittent Fasting For Bodybuilder & Athletes

It is quite obvious that someone who is overweight will benefit from intermittent fasting. Also, this book has shown that intermittent fasting has real benefits in many different ways for those who wish to be healthier and live longer as well as those who want to lose weight.

However, what about an athlete who needs to be in peak condition?

Will this put his or her body under high stress as a result of heavy training and intense competition?

Research has shown that the effect of intermittent fasting on athletes who were training hard was very beneficial. The research was on athletes who were training hard and whose intake of calories were about 3000 per day for each of the athletes. The ratio of macronutrients was 55% from carbohydrate, 24% from fats and 21% from protein. No snacks were allowed in between meals, although the athletes were given 20 grams of whey protein after each workout. There was a feast/fast pattern each day.

By this research, a 16/8 -12/12 protocol was determined as best for athletes involved in heavy training in preference to the 18/6-20/4 protocols. So far there has been no research that I am aware of on the 5:2 diet for athletes doing intense training. It would be interesting to see if there were similar results.

What is quite clear is that it is vital for athletes doing heavy training to make sure that they do not have a low carbohydrate diet and that they get plenty of protein.

Chapter 7: How to Get Started on Intermittent Fasting

Intermittent fasting is not just a diet, in the long run; it does seem like a lifestyle choice. This diet neither places any restriction on the calories consumed nor does it cut certain food groups out of your regular diet. Instead, intermittent fasting restricts the hours during the day in which you can eat. Intermittent fasting alternates between periods of eating and fasting. The fasting period usually includes the time spent sleeping and all those hours during which you aren't allowed to eat. There are different variations of this diet. As mentioned in the earlier chapters, this diet can be successfully paired with exercise or calorie reduction for weight loss or muscle gain. Depending on your needs and requirements, this diet can be easily altered. In this chapter, you will learn the way in which you can adopt an intermittent fasting protocol into your daily life. There are three steps for easing yourself into this diet, and they have been discussed as follows.

Planning Your Fast

Always consult your medical practitioner before starting this diet. You may even want to talk to a nutritionist before you get started with this diet. Weigh in the pros and cons of this diet and inform the doctor about any pre-existing medical conditions. It is important that you consult your doctor because this diet can cause a significant change in your metabolism. If you are pregnant or aren't feeling well, then don't start this diet. All those who have type-1 diabetes shouldn't follow this diet because it will be difficult to maintain the necessary insulin levels with a strict fasting protocol.

Select an eating schedule that is sustainable: When you are thinking about implementing this diet, you will have to go for prolonged periods of time without food (this can last for a couple of hours to as long as 24 hours) before you get to eat anything. Intermittent fasting is an effective way to lose weight, regulate your eating habits and keep an eye on what you are eating. It is important that the schedule you have opted for is easy to maintain. You will have to ease yourself into this diet slowly. Start by having two meals a day instead of three, and set a time frame within which you are supposed to have your last meal.

Choose and maintain a minimum calorie requirement. Restrict the number of times you snack in a day. Each snack shouldn't be more than 20-30 calories (have a few sticks of celery or carrot, a portion of/or an apple, a few raisins, or an ounce of chicken or fish) until your fast comes to an end. A couple of the viable methods that you can choose from are as follows.

One meal window would mean that you would have to fast for 23 hours daily and choose a one-hour window during which you can eat a healthy meal. A two-meal window would mean that you could have two meals per day. The first one could be at noon and the next one at 6 or 7 in the evening. Then you will fast for the next 16 hours or so and have your next meal the following day. You can also skip a day and not eat on particular days. Depending upon your convenience, select a plan that is viable and sustainable for you.

Gradually reduce your calorie consumption. If you are used to having 2000-3000 calories per day, then you can start by cutting down the calories slowly. You can start by cutting down the calories you consume to 1500-2000 per day. Create a diet plan for yourself that will include healthy carbs, complex carbs, and some essential fats. Regardless of the calorie limit, you have set for yourself and the method you have opted for, you will have to consume your daily calories within the selected time frame. Calorie reduction becomes easier due to the time-constraint placed on the feeding time.

Don't make any dramatic alternations to your diet. While following intermittent fasting, you aren't required to cut out any food groups from your daily diet (for instance, you don't have to worry about giving up carbs or fats). The only condition is that you should have healthy and well-balanced meals without exceeding 2000 calories per day. The only thing that this diet changes will be your eating schedule. A diet that is well balanced will have healthy proteins, lots of vegetables, some fruit, and a moderate dose of carbs.

Following a Fasting Schedule

Easing into the diet. If you aren't used to fasting, then this particular diet might be quite a change for your system. It is bound to surprise your system and your appetite. Slowly transition yourself into this diet. You can start by increasing the gap between your meals or start by taking a day off from eating each week. This will help your body to get accustomed to fasting and help in eliminating or reducing uncomfortable side effects like headaches, low blood pressure, and fatigue. During the initial stages of this diet, you can have a couple of light snacks during the fasting period like a handful of nuts, some cheese or some light protein. Make sure that these snacks are less than 100 calories each. These snacks will not obstruct the effectiveness of this diet, at least not initially. Once you start getting used to this, you can start reducing the number of snacks you have. Start altering your diet gradually, so that it doesn't come as a shock to your system. For instance, start by limiting and then eliminating processed foods (includes processed meats) and sugary foods (like soda) slowly.

Have your last non-fasting meal. Resist the temptation of having lots of junk and processed foods for your last meal before you start the intermittent fast. Have lots of fresh vegetables, fruit, and lots of protein to make sure that your energy levels don't plummet. For instance, the "last" meal could consist of chicken breast, a portion of garlic bread and some salad with a hearty dressing. Some people tend to binge before starting this diet. This means that once they start their diet, their body will be busy digesting the food from the previous meal instead of getting used to the "fasting" phase. Have a well-balanced meal before you start fasting. This means that you shouldn't fill your tummy with food that's rich in carbs or sugar, since the chances of feeling hungry after such a meal are quite high. Have plenty of protein and healthy fats during your scheduled meal. Have fewer carbs, but compensate for this with plenty of protein and fats.

Fast during your sleeping hours. If you make sure that your fasting period coincides with your sleeping schedule, you can at least keep your mind off any hunger pangs in the middle of the fasting period. Make sure that you are getting an average of 8 hours sleep per night. Doing this will make it easier to fast, and you will not feel like you are depriving yourself of food. Think of the first meal that you have after breaking your fast as your reward for getting through the fasting period. You are bound to be hungry after fasting, so make sure that you have a full meal.

Keep yourself thoroughly hydrated. Regardless of whether it is your fasting or eating period, make sure that your body is hydrated. It is important that you keep yourself thoroughly hydrated, even more so when you are fasting for making sure that your body is functioning properly. You can have any beverage that doesn't have any calories in it. Keeping yourself hydrated will also help in keeping hunger at bay. You can have herbal teas, black tea or coffee, and plenty of water!

Losing Weight Through This Diet

Setting a weight loss goal. Intermittent fasting is a great way to lose weight. The reduction in the daily intake of calories automatically leads to weight loss since your body starts to burn its fat reserves for producing energy. A reduction in the time spent eating will help in the shedding of excess body fat by speeding up your metabolism. This diet also helps in reduction of inflammation in the body. The first thing you need to do to lose weight with this diet is to set a weight loss goal for yourself. The motivation to keep going improves when you have a goal to work towards. This will provide you with the extra mental strength that's necessary to keep fasting. The reduction in the time spent eating will help in reducing the chances of gaining weight as well.

Build muscle mass while fasting. Intermittent fasting is a dieting protocol that allows you to build muscle. Plan your day in such a manner that you can squeeze in some exercise right before your first meal of the day or between two meals if need be. Your body will be able to burn the calories efficiently. So, make sure that you have about 60% of your daily calories right after your workout. To maintain the health and improving the muscle mass, make sure that the number of calories consumed doesn't go below ten calories per pound of your body weight. For instance, an individual who weighs around 170 pounds will need to have at least 1700 calories per day to get lean. Starvation would be of no help. It might just cause more harm than any good.

Your exercise style should meet your desired body goal. The type of exercise that you perform while on this diet will depend on the results you desire. If you are just trying to shed a few kilos, then aerobic exercises and cardio will do. If you are seeking to build your muscle mass, then anaerobic exercises like weight training will be required. Aerobic exercises can be performed for longer than anaerobic exercises. Depending on your fitness and weight loss goals, you should select the kind of exercises you will want to indulge in.

Chapter 8: Little Tricks and Strategies to Not Die When Fasting

Well, now that you know what intermittent fasting is all about, the next logical step is to get started with the fasting protocol of your choice. Here are a couple of tricks that will come in handy when you initiate your intermittent fasting diet and your body tries to pull you out of it.

- Whenever you feel hunger or a hunger pang strikes you, it will take about 15 minutes to pass. So, take a couple of deep breaths, have a glass of water or you can have some herbal tea to just take the edge off. Let your hunger pang pass you by and don't give into it.

- When you have to break your fast, try to resist temptation of gorging on food the minute your fasting period is over. Let that phase of intense hunger pass you by or at least ease up a little before you start eating. Also, when you start eating, eat slowly. Make sure that you are sitting down while eating. Chew your food carefully, relish the flavor, and don't just stuff yourself with food. Avoid all forms of distractions when it's your eating time. Keep your phone away, don't surf the Internet, and don't watch TV. Enjoy the food you are eating. Think about the textures and flavors. Mindless eating often tends to result in overeating. This needs to be avoided, or you will simply be undoing all the effort you put into it while fasting. Practice mindful eating.

- Have foods that are rich in nutrients. This is the most ideal way to go about having your meal, even more so when you are fasting for prolonged periods of time. Your main aim when your fast ends is to nourish your body with wholesome food. Have lots of protein, vegetables, and nuts. Have some dessert if you feel like it, but do so after you have had the food that you should have.

Nutrition needs to be a priority. By practicing mindful eating, you will be able to tell when you are feeling full. Don't keep eating because there is more food or because you have been fasting all day long. This will just undo all the effort that you have put into fasting.

- Keep yourself busy. If you are occupied with some work, you will not sit and think about how hungry you are or what you would like to eat. The possibility of thinking about food increases when you are idle. Get fully involved in whatever you are doing. Do your best to keep yourself occupied and your mind off food. Get done with the majority of your work before sundown. Your energy levels are bound to be higher during morning hours than in the evening or afternoon. So, get your work done quickly.

- Once your body gets used to burning stored fat to generate energy, you can start incorporating a little bit of high-intensity workout into your daily schedule. It is even better if you manage to do this while you are fasting. This will enable and encourage your body to start burning stored fat to provide your body with energy. Exercising will also help in keeping your hunger at bay. However, this isn't recommended if you are new to fasting or you have just shifted to intermittent fasting from a diet that is rich in sugar and carbs. Over exertion will make you feel light headed and shaky, so proceed with caution and don't stretch yourself beyond what your body can handle. Make sure that your body is thoroughly hydrated even while exercising.

- During the initial phase of this diet, it is quite likely that you might tend to overeat when you break your fast. This isn't a major issue and it will resolve itself in a couple of days. Once your body gets used to fasting, this will not happen frequently. Even after fasting for 16 hours, you will be able to eat a normal-sized meal without overeating.

- Whenever you are hungry during the eating period, make sure that you are eating something. Calories do matter, but remember that you are eating so that you can get through the fasting period. If you feel hungry even after eating a meal, have a snack. It is okay to eat and don't worry about it.

- Whenever you feel like eating something during your fasting window, you can keep hunger at bay by following delayed gratification. If you feel like having some cereal, then simply tell yourself "not now, maybe later." This will help to take your mind off things without causing any trouble. You can make a list of stuff that you would like to eat once your fast ends.

- If you want to, you can break up your week with longer and shorter fasts instead of just sticking to one type of fast. If you feel like, you can do two 24-

hour fasts in a week and on the other days you can follow the lean gains model. This will help to make sure that your calorie intake is kept in check.

- It gets easier to follow intermittent fasting if you make sure that you are having high-quality carbs or complex carbs (they tend to have a lower glycemic index and help in maintaining your blood sugar within normal limit). This will also enable your body to start burning all the stored fat to provide you with energy. Once your blood sugar level is stabilized, the chances of feeling hungry due to a drop in the blood sugar can be avoided.

- Make sure that you are having your last meal at least a couple of hours before going to bed. If you have had sufficient food during your eating window, then you shouldn't feel hungry before sleeping. Even if you do, this hunger will be gone by the time you are up in the morning.

- Getting sufficient sleep should be a priority. Lack of sleep will make you feel hungry, more than usual. This will also disrupt your entire day. It is not just about getting sleep, the quality of sleep matters as well. It is not only important for maintaining your overall health, but it is an important aspect of weight-loss as well. Two main reasons that obstruct weight loss are lack of sleep and stress.

- At times, it is okay to end your fast before the fasting period actually ends. Don't let this stress you out. If you feel extremely hungry, it is okay to break your fast. However, don't let this become a habit. Stressing yourself out won't do you any good and you will simply end up sabotaging your own diet. Even if you deviate from your diet once in a while, it is okay.

- The type of food and its quality are more important than the frequency of meals when it comes to maintaining the required nutrition, overall health, and fat loss. No two individuals are alike. An intermittent fasting protocol that works for one person might not work for someone else. The only way to find a method that works best for you is by experimentation. Intermittent fasting does help in simplifying your day, provided you do a couple of things beforehand. You should always have your post-fast meals ready for when your fast ends. This will save you the trouble of having to decide what to eat and if you decide in advance, it is likely that you will have a healthy meal.

Some Final Words

Thank you again for reading this book! All the information that you will need about intermittent fasting has been provided in this book. Fasting for a prolonged period has multiple benefits, and it will improve the overall functioning of your body. The two cardinal rules of intermittent fasting are - eat only during the feeding window and make sure that the food is healthy and wholesome.

While fasting, make sure that your body is thoroughly hydrated and you are having plenty of fluids. There are different variations of this diet and try them until you find one that works the best for you. If you are okay with the idea of fasting for 24 hours, then you can select the alternate day fasting method. If you are okay with the idea of fasting daily, then you can opt for the 16/8 method or the warrior diet. Select a diet plan based on your needs and convenience.

Make sure that you consult your physician or medical practitioner before you get started with this diet. Do plenty of research before you select a method, eat the right food, and include some form of exercise into your daily routine. You will be able to see a positive difference in no time. By following intermittent fasting, you will be able to attain your health and weight loss goals.

I hope this book proved to be informative. If you liked this book and enjoyed reading it, then please review it on Amazon. I'll be glad to hear your feedback.

Start now, act and I'm sure you'll be glad you did.

Good luck fasting!

9 781976 308000